One Day at a Time
Food Journal
&
Hunger and Fullness Monitor

Real World Nutrition
www.realworldnutrition.org
Rebekah Hennes, R.D.

Published and distributed in the United States by:
CCH Services, Inc.
Real World Nutrition, 8862 Earhart Ave
Los Angeles, CA 90045
(562)895-0682 ● (310)861-5053 fax

The author does not dispense any medical advice or prescribe the use of any technique without the advice of a physician, either directly or indirectly. The intent of the author is to offer you advice on how to learn about and document your food intake and physical hunger and fullness cues. In the event that you use any of the information in this book for yourself, which is your constitutional right, the author and the publisher assume no responsibility for your actions.

Library of Congress Cataloging-in-Publication Data

Mardis, Rebekah

One Day at a Time,
Food Journal and Hunger and Fullness Monitor / Rebekah Mardis
ISBN # 0-9768383-1-1
ISBN 13 # 978-0-9768383-1-9

1. Health
2. Nutrition

ISBN # 0-9768383-1-1
ISBN 13 # 978-0-9768383-1-9

1st Printing, April 2007
2nd Printing, October 2007

Printed by: RJ Communications, LLC
New York, NY

CONTENTS

Introduction

INTRODUCTION

By recognizing and honoring your hunger and fullness cues, you will be listening to your body. Learning how to listen to your body without judgment is the key to normal eating and maintaining a healthy body weight. The more time that you take to listen to your body, the more obvious your hunger and fullness cues will become.

Chronic dieting affects a person's ability to recognize hunger and fullness. If you have a history of dieting, you will want to work through your food issues with a dietitian and a therapist so that you will be able to accurately listen to your body. In the past, if you restricted nutrients (fat, protein, or carbohydrates) your body may be presently "deprived", either nutritionally or experientially. Your body may have adapted to this deprivation by accepting a constant low-grade hunger as homeostasis. This constant hunger will persist until your body and psyche no longer feel "deprived".

If you are currently restricting nutrients, it will be difficult for you to recognize the actual sensation of satiety. Even if you eat a meal that has adequate calories, your body may not be getting the specific building blocks that it needs to perform its daily functions. If this is the case, you will not experience an actual satisfied feeling after eating a restrictive meal. For example, if you were to eat a large salad you may feel physically full and yet not satisfied.

The only way for you to really know if your body is getting enough calories, as well as the specific types of food that it needs, is to begin using a food journal to gain insight into your food intake. After you have kept a record of your food intake, for a week or two, you can ask for advice from a dietitian, who will then have the information contained in your completed food journal to be able to offer you suggestions, as appropriate.

By learning how to recognize and respond to your hunger, fullness, and cravings, you will not only be giving your body the food that it needs, you will also be eating the amounts of food that your body requires to maintain a healthy body weight.

WHICH FOOD JOURNAL TO USE

In this book, there are two variations of a food journal, as well as one hunger and fullness monitor. You can read the descriptions and the examples for each, and determine which is best for you to use at the present time. At first, you may only want to write down what you are eating. If this is the case, use either the "Food Journal #1" (see page #14) or the "Hunger and Fullness Monitor and Food Journal #2" (see page #16).

On the other hand, if you are interested in learning how to recognize your hunger and fullness cues, as well as learning how your emotions play a role in your relationship with food, then you can use the "Hunger and Fullness Monitor and Food Journal #2" (see page #16) or the "Hunger and Fullness Monitor #3" (see page #18). Before you begin monitoring your hunger and fullness levels, you should read through the "Frequently Asked Questions and Concerns" chapter located at the back of this book to answer some of the questions that you may already have.

HOW TO MONITOR YOUR HUNGER AND FULLNESS

It may take time for you to recognize your hunger and fullness sensations. You will need to be very honest with yourself. You will also need to give yourself permission to feel hungry, to eat, and to feel satisfied without judging the sensations as good, bad, right, or wrong. At first, you may need to guess what your hunger and fullness cues are. You can solicit help with this experience by asking your friends or family how they recognize when they are hungry or full. Use the "Hunger / Satiety Scale" (which is located in the appendix) as a guide to help you become more aware of the physical cues that are related to hunger and fullness.

By monitoring your hunger and fullness levels, you will gain insight into when and why your hunger and fullness levels fluctuate. By recognizing your physical cues and documenting your eating experience without judgment, you may begin to see patterns. You may notice, as an example, that on Sundays you wait too long to eat, you get too hungry, eat too quickly, and then get too full. Or you may notice that you only eat every six hours, that you are hungrier than you think you are, or you may not yet be aware of what hunger feels like. On the other hand, you may notice that you are hungry every hour which is a clue that you may be restricting nutrients, or that you are coping with emotions by wanting to eat. You may document, in your food journal, you are only a little hungry but when you eat you may discover that you are actually very hungry.

EMOTIONS

It has been said that the stomach is the playground of the emotions. If this is so, your emotions play a role in your ability to recognize your hunger and fullness sensations. When you monitor your emotions, it is important to separate the emotion from the food that you eat or don't eat. If you eat a donut for breakfast, don't write: "I am furious and disappointed with myself for eating the donut". Instead, you want to document the emotion that you are feeling and separate it from the eating episode. "I am angry at my mother.", and "I ate a donut quickly".

Not only will you need to be able to separate the food that you eat from causing you to feel an emotion, you will also need to be able to recognize when an emotion is triggering you to eat or to restrict. Emotional and physical triggers to eat have very different causes, and yet they can feel similar. This is especially the case when you have made a habit of eating, or not eating, to cope with stress or emotions. In the appendix, there is a flow chart: "HUNGER- Physical vs. Emotional." This chart can help you figure out whether the hunger that you are experiencing is physical or emotional.

Also, in the appendix, there is an "Emotion List". You will want to orient yourself with this list, so that you are aware of the vast number of feelings that you could be experiencing at any given time. Please note, that here may be some emotions that you cannot currently recognize. By sharing your experience with a therapist you will be able to sort out your history, your tolerance threshold, and your ability to feel different emotions.

ONE DAY AT A TIME QUOTES

It is very helpful to practice being mindful while you journal your food intake and monitor your hunger, fullness, and emotions. If you allow your thoughts to be too far in the future, or too far in the past, it will be very difficult for you to recognize your body sensations in the moment. The quotes printed on each page of this book are to help you remember that you are living in, and working on, today. You will have to take baby steps and you will need to take your journey one day at a time. By doing so, you will definitely get wherever it is that you are headed.

"The baby rises to its feet, takes a step,
is overcome with triumph and joy-
and falls flat on its face.
It is a pattern for all that is to come!
But learn from the bewildered baby.
Lurch to your feet again. You'll make the sofa in the end."
~Pam Brown

Descriptions and Examples

Food Journal #1

Time	Emotions	Food	Urge B/R/P	Did B/R/P
6:00 AM	*I hate myself. Life sucks.*	*1 c cereal, 1c milk*	*no*	*no*
9:00 AM	*Life still sucks. Abandoned*	*¼ apple*	*no*	*no*
12:00 PM	*Guess it's time to eat. I can't study.*	*½ peanut butter sandwich*	*no*	*no*
3:00 PM	*Frustrated. I am thinking about food. I feel fat and ugly.*	*¼ apple*	*no*	*no*
6:00 PM	*Empty*	*Pot of coffee, salad with vinegar*	*no*	*no*
9:00 PM	*Depressed*	*Diet soda*	*no*	*no*

Date:_____

Food Journal #1

"Food Journal #1" has a column for you to write down what you eat and the time that you eat. This can be particularly helpful if you are seeing a dietitian who needs to know the foods, and the amount of food, that you are eating.

There is also a column for you to document what emotion you are feeling prior to eating. Remember that your emotion is not dictated by what you eat. Write down, instead, what you felt before eating. It may be a mood from the moment in general.

On the right side of this food journal, there are two columns for you to document eating disorder behavior. If you have an urge to binge, restrict, or purge you can note the urge in the second to the last column. In the last column you can document if you follow through on any of those behaviors. Also, if you do binge, it is very helpful and freeing, albeit challenging, to write down the foods that you eat during the binge.

Hunger and Fullness Monitor and Food Journal #2

Time	Emotion	Meal/Food	Hunger	Fullness
8:00 AM	Happy	Vente Latte	3	5
9:00 AM	Exilarated	Diet Soda	3	5
1:00 PM	Neutral	2 bean burritos, rice and beans, french fries double cheeseburger- I wanted to purge. I ate more. I have totally screwed up.	1	8
9:00 PM	Foolish	I am finally hungry again. Chicken noodle soup, bread with butter.	4	6
		Went to bed.		

Date:_____

Hunger and Fullness Monitor and Food Journal #2

The "Hunger and Fullness Monitor and Food Journal #2" is similar to the previous food journal. However, in this journal there is not a place for you to write down if you have an urge to binge, restrict, or purge. If you are working on changing any disordered eating behavior, and you do have the urge to use those behaviors, you can note this in the emotion section, so that you can discuss it with your dietitian without forgetting when it happened.

In this food journal, you have a choice to write down exactly what you eat for breakfast, or you can just write "breakfast" and not specify the individual food items (Meal/Food). In order to not specify the exact amounts and types of food that you are eating, you have to make sure that you are NOT restricting any type of food or nutrient.

On the other hand, if you are only working on recognizing the somatic cues of hunger and fullness, and how they relate to your emotions, you may not need to write down the foods that you eat. You can discuss your options further with your dietitian.

Hunger and Fullness Monitor #3

Time	Emotion	Meal	0	1	2	3	4	5	6	7	8	9
5:00pm	Angry	Dinner						X			X	
6:00pm	Frustrated	Snack					X				X	
7:00pm	Abandoned	Snack					X				X	
8:00am	Relieved	Breakfast				X		X				
10:00am	Neutral	Snack						X	X			
2:00pm	Overwhelmed	Lunch							X	X		
4:00pm	Paranoid	Snack							X	X		
6:00pm	Relieved	Dinner						X	X			
8:00am	Overwhelmed	Breakfast							X	X		
10:00am	Neutral	Snack						X	X			
2:00pm	Overwhelmed	Lunch							X	X		
4:00pm	Paranoid	Snack							X	X		
6:00pm	Relieved	Dinner						X	X			
8:00am	Overwhelmed	Breakfast							X	X		
10:00am	Neutral	Snack						X	X			
2:00pm	Overwhelmed	Lunch							X	X		
4:00pm	Paranoid	Snack							X	X		

Date:_____

The Hunger and Fullness Monitor #3

The "Hunger and Fullness Monitor #3" is a monitor, it is not a food journal. In this monitor, there is not space provided for you to write down the specific foods that you eat. Instead, it was designed to help you learn to recognize your hunger and fullness levels, as well as to help you become aware of how your emotions affect your hunger and fullness cues.

One example of when to use this monitor is if you are in an inpatient setting, and you know that your meals are not lacking any nutrients or calories. This monitor can also be used if you are at a point in recovery where you listen to your food cravings, you do not restrict, and you are ready to be mindful of how your emotions affect your ability to listen to your body.

Please notice that the hunger and fullness scale located in the appendix goes from a "0" to a "10". This monitor has a place for you to document your hunger and fullness level from a "0" to a "9". If you do get to a "10", you can: write an "X" on the outside of the table, document your experience in the "emotion" column, or document the incident at the bottom of the page (like a footnote).

Food Journal #1

Nothing is worth more than this day.--Johann Wolfgang von Goethe

Time	Emotion	Food	Urge B/R/ P	Did B/ R/ P

Date:_____

Normal day, let me be aware of the treasure you are. Let me learn from you, love you, bless you before you depart. Let me not pass you by in quest of some rare and perfect tomorrow. Let me hold you while I may, for it may not always be so. – Iorn

Time	Emotion	Food	Urge B/R/P	Did B/R/P

Date:_____

We are here and it is now.
Further than that, all human knowledge is moonshine.
--H. L. Mencken

Time	Emotion	Food	Urge B/R/ P	Did B/ R/ P

Date:_____

Never put off till tomorrow what you can do today.
You may enjoy doing it so much that you want to do it again.--Ross Perot

Time	Emotion	Food	Urge B/R/P	Did B/R/P

Date:_____

The more I give myself permission to live in the moment
and enjoy it without feeling guilty or judgmental about any other time,
the better I feel about the quality of my work.—Wayne Dyer

Time	Emotion	Food	Urge B/R/ P	Did B/ R/ P

Date:_____

Most of us think having a list of priorities is a sign of a motivated, serious person. But there is one essential flaw in this perspective. We are not guaranteed a future; and even if we were we could not live in it. All we have is now.—G. Lawrence-Ell

Time	Emotion	Food	Urge B/R/P	Did B/R/P

Date:_____

Make the best of today, for there is no tomorrow until after today.
--Liz Strehlow

Time	Emotion	Food	Urge B/R/ P	Did B/ R/ P

Date:_____

The more anger towards the past you carry in your heart, the less capable you are of loving in the present.--Barbara De Angelis

Time	Emotion	Food	Urge B/R/ P	Did B/ R/ P

Date:_____

Look not mournfully into the past, it comes not back again. Wisely improve the present, it is thine. Go forth to meet the shadowy future without fear and with a manly heart.--Henry Wadsworth Longfellow

Time	Emotion	Food	Urge B/R/P	Did B/R/P

Date:_____

Living in the moment means letting go of the past and not waiting for the future. It means living your life consciously, aware that each moment you breathe is a gift.
--Oprah Winfrey

Time	Emotion	Food	Urge B/R/ P	Did B/ R/ P

Date:_____

Light tomorrow with today!--Elizabeth Barrett Browning

Time	Emotion	Food	Urge B/R/P	Did B/R/P

Date:_____

Life is a succession of moments. To live each one is to succeed.--Coreta Kent

Time	Emotion	Food	Urge B/R/ P	Did B/ R/ P

Date:_____

Life is a great and wondrous mystery, and the only thing we know that we have for sure is what is right here right now. Don't miss it.--Leo Buscaglia

Time	Emotion	Food	Urge B/R/ P	Did B/ R/ P

Date:_____

Know the true value of time! Snatch, seize, and enjoy every moment of it.
No idleness, no procrastination.
Never put off until tomorrow what you can do today. --Philip Chesterfield

Time	Emotion	Food	Urge B/R/ P	Did B/ R/ P

Date:_____

I live now and only now, and I will do what I want to do this moment and not what I decided was best for me yesterday. --Hugh Prather

Time	Emotion	Food	Urge B/R/ P	Did B/ R/ P

Date:_____

One cannot change the past, but one can ruin the present by worrying over the future.--
Anonymous

Time	Emotion	Food	Urge B/R/P	Did B/R/P

Date:_____

I live a day at a time. Each day I look for a kernel of excitement. In the morning I say: "What is my exciting thing for today?" Then, I do the day. Don't ask me about tomorrow.--Barbara Jordan (Educom Review 2/17/98)

Time	Emotion	Food	Urge B/R/P	Did B/R/P

Date:_____

One day at a time--this is enough. Do not look back and grieve over the past, for it is gone; and do not be troubled about the future, for it has not yet come. Live in the present, and make it so beautiful that it will be worth remembering. -I. Scott Taylor

Time	Emotion	Food	Urge B/R/P	Did B/R/P

Date:_____

One of the most tragic things I know about human nature is that all of us tend to put off living. We are all dreaming of some magical rose garden over the horizon-instead of enjoying the roses blooming outside our windows today. —Dale Carnegie

Time	Emotion	Food	Urge B/R/ P	Did B/ R/ P

Date:_____

I shall make of this day--each moment of this day--a heaven on earth.
This is my day of opportunity.--Dan Custer

Time	Emotion	Food	Urge B/R/P	Did B/R/P

Date:_____

Don't look back on happiness, or dream of it in the future. You are only sure of today; do not let yourself be cheated out of it.--Henry Ward Beecher

Time	Emotion	Food	Urge B/R/P	Did B/R/P

Date:_____

The present time has one advantage over every other--it is our own.
--Charles Caleb Colton

Time	Emotion	Food	Urge B/R/ P	Did B/ R/ P

Date:_____

Reflect upon your present blessings, of which every man has plenty; not on your past misfortunes of which all men have some.--Charles Dickens

Time	Emotion	Food	Urge B/R/ P	Did B/ R/ P

Date:_____

Remember then: there is only one time that is important--Now! It is the most important time because it is the only time when we have any power.
--Leo Tolstoy ("Three Questions")

Time	Emotion	Food	Urge B/R/ P	Did B/ R/ P

Date:_____

Live only for the hour and its allotted work. Think not of the amount to be accomplished, the difficulties to be overcome, or the end to be attained, but set earnestly at the little task at your elbow, letting that be sufficient for the day. —Osler

Time	Emotion	Food	Urge B/R/P	Did B/R/P

Date:_____

The secret of health for both mind and body is not to mourn for the past,
nor to worry about the future,
but to live the present moment wisely and earnestly.—Buddha

	Emotion	Food	Urge B/R/ P	Did B/ R/ P

Date:_____

Make the best of today, for there is no tomorrow until after today.
--Liz Strehlow

Time	Emotion	Food	Urge B/R/P	Did B/R/P

Date:_____

Hunger and Fullness Monitor
&
Food Journal #2

One day at a time--this is enough. Do not look back and grieve over the past, for it is gone; and do not be troubled about the future, for it has not yet come. Live in the present, and make it so beautiful that it will be worth remembering. I. Scott Taylor

Time	Emotion	Meal/Food	Hunger	Fullness

Date:_____

She seems to have had the ability to stand firmly on the rock of her past while living completely and unregretfully in the present.--Madeleine L'Engle (The Summer of the Great-Grandmother)

Time	Emotion	Meal/Food	Hunger	Fullness

Date:_____

Some people are making such thorough preparation for rainy days that they aren't enjoying today's sunshine.--William Feather

Time	Emotion	Meal/Food	Hunger	Fullness

Date:_____

Nothing is worth more than this day.--Johann Wolfgang von Goethe

Time	Emotion	Meal/Food	Hunger	Fullness

Date:_____

I always feel sorry for people who think more about a rainy day ahead than sunshine today.--Rae Foley (*Suffer a Witch*)

Time	Emotion	Meal/Food	Hunger	Fullness

Date:_____

When one door closes another door opens; but we so often look so long and so regretfully upon the closed door, that we do not see the ones which open for us.
~Alexander Graham Bell

Time	Emotion	Meal/Food	Hunger	Fullness

Date:_____

Having spent the better part of my life trying either to relive the past or experience the future before it arrives, I have come to believe that in between these two extremes is peace. *~Author Unknown*

Time	Emotion	Meal/Food	Hunger	Fullness

Date:_____

Today a new sun rises for me; everything lives, everything is animated, everything seems to speak to me of my passion, everything invites me to cherish it...
--Anne de Lencios

Time	Emotion	Meal/Food	Hunger	Fullness

Date:_____

"Old times" never come back and I suppose it's just as well. What comes back is a new morning every day in the year, and that's better. ~George E. Woodberry

Time	Emotion	Meal/Food	Hunger	Fullness

Date:_____

People are always asking about the good old days.
I say, why don't you say the good now days? ~Robert M. Young

Time	Emotion	Meal/Food	Hunger	Fullness

Date:_____

No yesterdays are ever wasted for those who give themselves to today.
~Brendan Francis

Time	Emotion	Meal/Food	Hunger	Fullness

Date:_____

The past is a guidepost, not a hitching post.
~L. Thomas Holdcroft

Time	Emotion	Meal/Food	Hunger	Fullness

Date:_____

Time	Emotion	Meal/Food	Hunger	Fullness

Date:_____

True happiness is...to enjoy the present,
without anxious dependence upon the future.--Seneca

Time	Emotion	Meal/Food	Hunger	Fullness

Date:_____

Very strange is this quality of our human nature which decrees that unless we feel a future before us we do not live completely in the present.--Phillips Brooks

Time	Emotion	Meal/Food	Hunger	Fullness

Date:_____

Don't let yesterday use up too much of today. ~*Cherokee Indian Proverb*

Time	Emotion	Meal/Food	Hunger	Fullness

Date:_____

Yesterday is a canceled check; tomorrow is a promissory note; today is the only cash you have. Spend it wisely.--Anonymous

Time	Emotion	Meal/Food	Hunger	Fullness

Date:_____

If you are still talking about what you did yesterday, you haven't done much today.
~Author Unknown

Time	Emotion	Meal/Food	Hunger	Fullness

Date:_____

I have memories - but only a fool stores his past in the future.
~David Gerrold

Time	Emotion	Meal/Food	Hunger	Fullness

Date:_____

With the past, I have nothing to do; nor with the future. I live now.
~*Ralph Waldo Emerson*

Time	Emotion	Meal/Food	Hunger	Fullness

Date:_____

Yesterday's the past, tomorrow's the future, but today is a gift.
That's why it's called the present.--Bil Keane

Time	Emotion	Meal/Food	Hunger	Fullness

Date:_____

Yesterday is a canceled check; tomorrow is a promissory note; today is the only cash you have. Spend it wisely.--Anonymous

Time	Emotion	Meal/Food	Hunger	Fullness

Date:_____

We are here and it is now.
Further than that, all human knowledge is moonshine .--H. L. Mencken

Time	Emotion	Meal/Food	Hunger	Fullness

Date:_____

Very strange is this quality of our human nature which decrees that unless we feel a future before us we do not live completely in the present.--Phillips Brooks

Time	Emotion	Meal/Food	Hunger	Fullness

Date:_____

True happiness is...to enjoy the present,
without anxious dependence upon the future.--Seneca

Time	Emotion	Meal/Food	Hunger	Fullness

Date:_____

Tomorrow's life is too late. Live today.--Martial

Time	Emotion	Meal/Food	Hunger	Fullness

Date:_____

Today a new sun rises for me; everything lives, everything is animated,
everything seems to speak to me of my passion,
everything invites me to cherish it...--Anne de Lencios

Time	Emotion	Meal/Food	Hunger	Fullness

Date:_____

Some people are making such thorough preparation for rainy days that they aren't enjoying today's sunshine.--William Feather

Time	Emotion	Meal/Food	Hunger	Fullness

Date:_____

She seems to have had the ability to stand firmly on the rock of her past while living completely and un-regretfully in the present.
--Madeleine L'Engle (The Summer of the Great-Grandmother)

Time	Emotion	Meal/Food	Hunger	Fullness

Date:_____

The secret of health for both mind and body is not to mourn for the past, nor to worry about the future, but to live the present moment wisely and earnestly.--Buddha

Time	Emotion	Meal/Food	Hunger	Fullness

Date:_____

Remember then: there is only one time that is important--Now! It is the most important time because it is the only time when we have any power.
--Leo Tolstoy ("Three Questions")

Time	Emotion	Meal/Food	Hunger	Fullness

Date:_____

Reflect upon your present blessings, of which every man has plenty; not on your past misfortunes of which all men have some.--Charles Dickens

Time	Emotion	Meal/Food	Hunger	Fullness

Date:_____

The present time has one advantage over every other--it is our own.
--Charles Caleb Colton (Lacon)

Time	Emotion	Meal/Food	Hunger	Fullness

Date:_____

Hunger and Fullness Monitor #3

The secret of health for both mind and body is not to mourn for the past, nor to worry about the future, but to live the present moment wisely and earnestly- Buddha

Time	Emotion	Meal	0	1	2	3	4	5	6	7	8	9

Date:_____

One of the most tragic things I know about human nature is that all of us tend to put off living. We are all dreaming of some magical rose garden over the horizon-instead of enjoying the roses blooming outside our windows today.--Dale Carnegie

Time	Emotion	Meal	0	1	2	3	4	5	6	7	8	9

Date:_____

One day at a time--this is enough. Do not look back and grieve over the past, for it is gone; and do not be troubled about the future, for it has not yet come. Live in the present, and make it so beautiful that it will be worth remembering.-I. Scott Taylor

Time	Emotion	Meal	0	1	2	3	4	5	6	7	8	9

Date:_____

There is no distance on this earth as far away as yesterday.
~Robert Nathan, *So Love Returns*

Time	Emotion	Meal	0	1	2	3	4	5	6	7	8	9

Date:_____

One cannot change the past, but one can ruin the present
by worrying over the future.—*Anonymous*

Time	Emotion	Meal	0	1	2	3	4	5	6	7	8	9

Date:_____

Nothing is worth more than this day.--Johann Wolfgang von Goethe

Time	Emotion	Meal	0	1	2	3	4	5	6	7	8	9

Date:_____

Normal day, let me be aware of the treasure you are. Let me learn from you, love you, bless you before you depart. Let me not pass you by in quest of some rare and perfect tomorrow. Let me hold you while I may, for it may not always be so.-M. Iron

Time	Emotion	Meal	0	1	2	3	4	5	6	7	8	9

Date:_____

Never put off till tomorrow what you can do today.
You may enjoy doing it so much that you want to do it again.--Ross Perot

Time	Emotion	Meal	0	1	2	3	4	5	6	7	8	9

Date:_____

Most of us think having a list of priorities is a sign of a motivated, serious person. But there is one essential flaw in this perspective. We are not guaranteed a future; and even if we were we could not live in it. All we have is no.--George Lawrence-Ell

Time	Emotion	Meal	0	1	2	3	4	5	6	7	8	9

Date:_____

The most important revelation about the past stems from the realization that it is not important to try and get rid of it, but to realize that we are already, by definition, rid of it. The only reality is now.--George Lawrence-Ell

Time	Emotion	Meal	0	1	2	3	4	5	6	7	8	9

Date:_____

The more I give myself permission to live in the moment and enjoy it without feeling guilty or judgmental about any other time, the better I feel about the quality of my work.--Wayne Dyer

Time	Emotion	Meal	0	1	2	3	4	5	6	7	8	9

Date:_____

The more anger towards the past you carry in your heart,
the less capable you are of loving in the present.--Barbara De Angelis

Time	Emotion	Meal	0	1	2	3	4	5	6	7	8	9

Date:_____

Make the best of today, for there is no tomorrow until after today.
--Liz Strehlow

Time	Emotion	Meal	0	1	2	3	4	5	6	7	8	9

Date:_____

Make it a rule of life never to regret and never to look back. Regret is an appalling waste of energy, you can't build on it it's only good for wallowing in.
--Katherine Mansfield

Time	Emotion	Meal	0	1	2	3	4	5	6	7	8	9

Date:_____

Look not mournfully into the past, it comes not back again. Wisely improve the present, it is thine. Go forth to meet the shadowy future without fear and with a manly heart.--Henry Wadsworth Longfellow

Time	Emotion	Meal	0	1	2	3	4	5	6	7	8	9

Date:_____

Living in the moment means letting go of the past and not waiting for the future.
It means living your life consciously, aware that each moment you breathe is a gift.
--Oprah Winfrey

Time	Emotion	Meal	0	1	2	3	4	5	6	7	8	9

Date:_____

Light tomorrow with today!--Elizabeth Barrett Browning

Time	Emotion	Meal	0	1	2	3	4	5	6	7	8	9

Date:_____

Frequently Asked
Questions and Concerns

FREQUENTLY ASKED QUESTIONS AND CONCERNS
The answers are on the following pages.

Deprivation/Restricting
- What do I need to know before I eat a previously forbidden food?
- When I try to eat a regular sized meal I am still hungry. What should I do?
- I am waiting to eat until I am ravenous, and then I feel out of control.

Emotions
- How do I know if I am emotionally eating?
- When I get upset, I do not want to eat.

Fullness
- I am a little over-full after eating a special meal.
- I just ate and I am uncomfortably full. What do I do?
- I am consistently over-eating. What should I do?

Hunger
- I am hungry all the time.
- I have no idea if I am hungry or full.

Medication
- Medication and Hunger

Purging
- Right after I purge I am very hungry. Why?

Types of food
- Fat, Hunger, and Satiety
- I am a vegetarian. Does protein really matter?
- I am scared to eat fat. Does eating fat really matter?

Deprivation/Restricting

- What do I need to know before I eat a previously forbidden food?

First, make sure that you are not too hungry before you eat. If you are at a "5" on the hunger and fullness scale, it is an appropriate time to eat your previously forbidden food. Please note, because you have deprived yourself of this particular food, it has probably become "special" to you. When a food becomes "special", and you finally let yourself eat it, you will likely get overfull (an "8" on the hunger and fullness scale). If this happens, the only consequence you have, is that you will be full longer than you would have been if you had stopped eating when you were at a satisfied level of a "6" or a "7". In order for you to be able to stop at a satisfied fullness level, you will need to not restrict your self from this food ever again. The more that you give yourself permission to eat, the less "special" your favorite foods will become, and then you will be able to stop eating when you are satisfied.

- When I try to eat a regular-sized meal, I am still hungry. What should I do?

You have a few options. You can eat until you are at a "7" on the hunger and fullness scale, and tell yourself that you will eat again when you are at a "4". You may also try eating a larger volume of food, more protein, or more fat. Or you could find non-food activities to occupy your time after eating. With time, your stomach's response to food will become more natural.

For your information, the stomach does not shrink or stretch but it is "volume sensitive". If your stomach has gotten used to being filled with large volumes of food then it may not send your brain appropriate signals of fullness. Until your stomach gets used to eating a smaller volume of food, you may just need to eat more often. You will also want to confirm with your dietitian that you are not restricting any nutrient, and that you are not emotionally eating.

Also, if you binge and purge, your body has probably gotten used to needing the stomach to be very full in order for the body to have enough nutrients to work with. For example, if you were to binge on 10,000 calories, then purge 9,000 of those calories, your body has 1,000 calories left to work with. Therefore, your body learns that is has to be 10,000 calories full in order for the body to actually process 1,000 calories. Your stomach gets used to a large volume of food equaling a smaller amount of usable energy. So, when you eat a small meal, the stomach may not send the same "satisfied" feedback to the brain, and you will think that you are still hungry. After a few weeks of consistently eating smaller meals, your stomach will send your brain more accurate feedback. In the meantime, you need to be patient and allow at least twenty minutes post-meal for your body to recognize that you have eaten an adequate number of calories.

- I am waiting to eat until I am ravenous, and then I feel out of control.

In order for you to feel like you have some control over your eating you have to eat before you get to a hunger level of "2" and for some people "3". If you allow yourself to get to a starving point prior to eating, you will experience what feels like a binge (eating quickly, feeling out of control or eating large amounts of food). If you allow yourself to be at a starving point for several hours, you may transition to fasting numbness, no longer crave food, or have any hunger sensations. You must remember that if you do allow yourself to get to a hunger level of "0" that you are causing your metabolism to slow down.

Emotions

- How do I know if I am emotionally eating?

Emotional eating is eating when the body is not hungry, eating to decrease emotional sensations, or eating to distract your self from thoughts or feelings. It is filling your body with food instead of feeling your emotions. Use your food journal and monitor to document the emotions that you are experiencing prior to eating. You can use the flow chart (in the appendix) to help you differentiate physical and emotional hunger. If you do find that you are emotionally eating, the next step is for you to practice alternative coping methods. The "gold-standard" method is dealing with your emotions head-on such as experiencing the emotion, writing about it, or talking about it. The second method entails doing some nurturing activity such as taking a bath or listening to music. The third coping method is to distract your self from the situation by doing an activity such as reading a book or watching a movie. Coping with an emotion or situation without using food can be similar to that of breaking any addiction. It is not easy.

- When I get upset, I do not want to eat.

Emotional restricting is similar to emotional eating. It has different means but the same end. If you are faced with a challenging situation, or emotion, and you do not eat or you eat very little as a way to cope with, or numb, your feelings then you are using restricting as a coping method. If this has become a habit for you, you will need to learn to separate your body cues from your emotions, and you will need to eat even if you are upset.

Fullness

- I am a little over-full after eating a special meal.

It is perfectly normal to get a little over-full on occasion. You will want to tune back into your hunger level as soon as you can without guilt, so that you do not feel the need to "finish the job" by eating more and /or purging.

- I just ate and I am uncomfortably full. What do I do?

Nothing, just wait. You will get hungry again, but it will take longer for this to happen. It is like you put a quarter into a parking meter instead of a dime. You just have more time to do other activities before you come back to feed the meter.

- I am consistently over-eating. What should I do?

Check in with yourself to see if you are emotionally eating, and learn other coping skills. If you consistently over-eat, then you will gain weight. But, if you get overfull less than twenty percent of the time your weight will probably not be affected. If your weight does go up because you get too full, too often, your weight will go back down after you have perfected your ability to stop eating at a satisfied level. You must be patient with the learning process.

Hunger

- I am hungry all the time.

If you are malnourished, underweight, or have been dieting you may experience a constant hunger sensation due to your body wanting to either gain weight, or to take in adequate nutrients such as protein, carbohydrates, or fat. It is not uncommon for you to feel like you want to overeat, or even experience overeating after dieting. This extreme hunger will decrease once you are back to your natural set-point weight, and are eating enough food so that your body does not react as if it is being starved.

- I have no idea if I am hungry or full.

You will usually begin to monitor your hunger and fullness levels inaccurately. You may think that you are very full when you eat a challenging food, or you may believe that you are full all of the time. It is important that you see a dietitian who can help you sort out your distorted translation of body cues. A dietitian will help you recognize what body sensations indicate that you are hungry and full. For example, if you think that you are at a "5", and you believe that you are not hungry prior to eating a meal, but you also are preoccupied with food, you have a headache, or you are feeling irritable, you are actually at a "2" on the hunger and fullness scale. On the other hand, if you believe that you are at an "8", but you are not uncomfortably full, then you are actually at a "6" on the hunger and fullness scale. As you can see, you will need some help understanding your hunger and fullness cues.

Medication

- Medication and Hunger

Some psychiatric medications trigger abnormal hunger and fullness signals. It is important for you to discuss your concerns with your psychiatrist, and to let your dietitian know what medications you are taking.

Purging

- Right after I purge I am very hungry. Why?

When you binge, insulin is dumped into the bloodstream. When you purge, some insulin stays in the veins to break down the glucose from the binge, and take it into the body for use. Because purging removes some of the food that the insulin was prepared to work on, the remaining insulin drops the blood sugar even lower which will cause you to feel hungry, and may trigger an episode of hypoglycemia. This is one of the causes of the continuous binge-purge-binge-purge cycle.

Types of food

- Fat, Hunger, and Satiety

Another factor contributing to your ability to stop eating when you are at a satisfied level has to do with your intake of fat, protein, and carbohydrate. You must be eating an adequate amount of fat and protein in order to feel satisfied. If you do not provide your body with the food that it needs you will experience a constant hunger. Also, you may not even recognize that you are hungry, because you are not able to recognize a fullness sensation for comparison. Some people describe this feeling as being constantly agitated.

When you add a significant amount of fat to your diet (approximately 30% or greater), you will be able to recognize satiety. After that, you will be able to differentiate hunger from fullness.

- I am a vegetarian. Does protein really matter?

Absolutely! Many people say that once they eat enough protein (3-4oz meat at a meal) they recognize being satisfied for a longer period of time. You will want to ask your dietitian if you are getting enough protein…especially if you are a vegetarian.

- I am scared to eat fat. Does eating fat really matter?

You bet. You may think that you cannot control yourself around carbohydrates, but the truth may be that you don't eat enough fat. Contemplate this exaggerated example: if a slice of bread contains 1 gram of fat, your body needs 60 grams, and you refuse to eat foods that have a high amount of fat in them, your body will not let you rest until it triggers you to eat 60 slices of bread just for the fat (6,000 calories). As contrast, if you ate 4 slices of bread with peanut butter (1/3 cup) you will eat far less calories because you will eat less than 60 slices of bread to ingest 60 grams of fat (approximately 1,000 calories total).

By restricting fat, you are causing your body to go on a hunt for inefficient sources of fat, and you will end up eating more calories in the process. Trying to replace fat with carbohydrates is like trying to give a car only gas when it is low on oil. Your best bet is to give yourself permission to eat all foods, and trust that your body will tell you what food it needs, when it needs it.

Some of the information in this section is taken from:
Reiff, DW, KKL Reiff. Eating Disorders: Nutrition therapy in the recovery process. Aspen Publishers, 1998.

Tribole, E, E Resch. Intuitive Eating: A revolutionary program that works. 2ⁿᵈ ed. New York: St. Martin's Griffin, 2003.

Appendix

#	HUNGER AND FULLNESS SCALE
10	Binge fullness. Sick feeling with stomach and back pain
9	"Thanksgiving Fullness". You need to unzip your pants in order to be comfortable.
8	Uncomfortable fullness that comes along with eating more than usual.
7	Fullness that allows you to leave the table without looking back. You may be bored of all of your food including the sweet taste. You are still not physically uncomfortable but you may not be totally comfortable.
6	Comfortable fullness that results in a satisfied feeling within ½ hour. Stop here and you will be satisfied for 3-4 hours.
5	Satisfied feeling that allows for more to be eaten.
4	Your senses indicate that you are hungry. Food looks good and tastes good. You may not know that you are hungry until you taste the food.
3	Stomach is empty and may growl. Need to eat soon.
2	Headache, irritable, tired, weak, light-headed, preoccupation with food. You may want to order everything and have a difficult time choosing what to order.
1	Starving point where you are ravenous for food "eating disorder hunger".
0	Fasting numbness that is felt when food is no longer craved.

EMOTION LIST

SAD	HAPPY	ANGRY	AFRAID
Abandoned	Amazed	Abused	Ambivalent
Agonized	Amused	Aggressive	Anxious
Apologetic	Calm	Alienated	Apprehensive
Burdened	Cherished	Angry	Bewildered
Desperate	Comfortable	Apathetic	Cautious
Disappointed	Confident	Appalled	Confused
Discouraged	Content	Blamed	Cowardly
Distant	Determined	Bitter	Disoriented
Disregarded	Delighted	Bored	Fearful
Embarrassed	Eager	Controlled	Frantic
Empty	Ecstatic	Disapproving	Frightened
Foolish	Exilarated	Disgusted	Hesitant
Forgotten	Free	Enraged	Insecure
Grief	Fulfilled	Envious	Panicked
Hopeless	Happy	Exasperated	Paranoid
Humiliated	Hopeful	Frustrated	Perplexed
Hurt	Important	Furious	Puzzled
Hysterical	Joyous	Guilty	Restless
Impotent	Loving	Hostile	Scared
Isolated	Loose	Horrified	Suspicious
Jinxed	Mellow	Impatient	Threatened
Lonely	Mischievious	Indifferent	Timid
Lost	Nurturing	Irritated	Torn
Miserable	Optimistic	Lethargic	Uncertain
Neglected	Peaceful	Manipulated	
Overlooked	Playful	Negative	
Regretful	Protective	Ornery	
Rejected	Proud	Resentful	
Upset	Relieved	Shocked	
Withdrawn	Respected	Smothered	
Worthless	Satisfied	Stubborn	
Vulnerable	Sympathetic	Victimized	

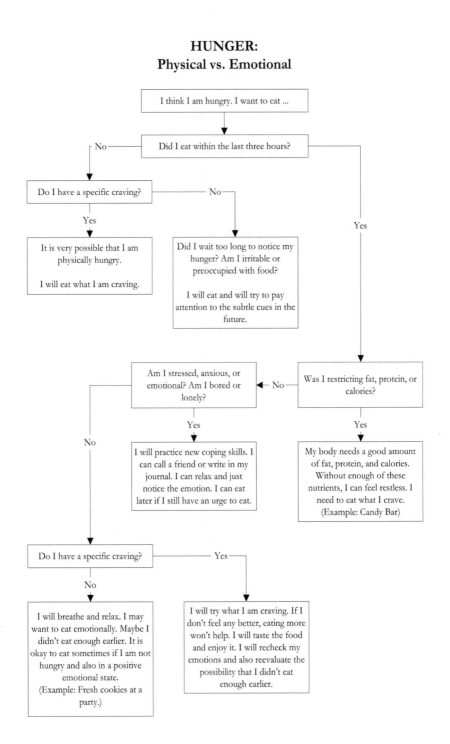

Look to this day,
For it is life, the very life of life.
In its brief course lie all the verities and realities of your existence;
the bliss of growth, the glory of action, the splendor of beauty.

For yesterday is but a dream
And tomorrow is only a vision,
But today well lived makes
every yesterday a dream of happiness
and every tomorrow a vision of hope.

Look well, therefore to this day,
such is the salutation of the dawn.--The Sufi, 1200 BC

Author: Rebekah Hennes, R.D.

Rebekah Hennes is a consulting Dietitian at the Eating Disorder Center of California and is in private practice in Brentwood, California. She recently edited and co-authored a new book entitled "Real World Recovery - Intuitive Food Program Curriculum for the Treatment of Eating Disorders" and authored "Return to Health", a guidebook for people with eating disorders. She was a contributor to the "Eating Disorder Sourcebook", 2nd Edition, and a reviewer of the American Dietetic Association position paper on Eating Disorders. Rebekah pioneered the Intuitive Food Program at the Center for Change in 1999.

You can reach Rebekah at: **rebekah@realworldnutrition.org.** For more information, please visit the Real World Nutrition website at: **www.realworldnutrition.org.**

●

Cover Art by: Coburn Hawk

Coburn Hawk is a Los Angeles based artist who creates "non-traditional Portraits." The finished Oil Paintings are snapshots of the subject's 'Spirit' (or that which is eternal in all of us.) After an in depth interview with each individual, the artist creates a representational piece not only of the person as they are now, but their larger purpose. It is a snapshot of the difference that individual makes on the world. The artist has become very adept at seeing this vision, even when the subject does not.

Parties interested in licensing existing artworks, limited run Giclee prints, Gallery exhibitions, or personal commissions may contact the artist through his website, **www.coburnhawk.com.**